BodyBuilding Diet:

For Women Over 40

By

Ann .D. Tijerina

by any means, including photocopying, recording, or other electronic or mechanical methods, without the prior written permission of the publisher, except in the case of brief quotations embodied in critical reviews and certain other noncommercial uses permitted by copyright law.

Copyright © (Dr. Susan M. Thomas), (2023).

Table of Content

Chapter 1: Understanding Body Building Diet for Women over 40

Introduction

Chapter 5: Staying on Track and Adapting to Changes

5.1 Staying Motivated and Accountable

5.2 Tracking Progress

5.3 Adjusting Diet and Exercise Routine

5.4 Adapting to Changes and Setbacks

Introduction

This book is explicitly intended to assist ladies north of 40 with accomplishing their lifting weights objectives through a legitimate and powerful eating regimen plan.

As ladies age, their body goes through many changes. It becomes more earnestly to fabricate and keep up with bulk, and weight gain becomes simpler. Be that as it may, with the right eating routine and exercise, ladies more than 40 can in any case accomplish their weight training objectives and keep a sound physical make-up. This book will zero in on the dietary part of working out for ladies north of 40 and give point by point direction on the most proficient method to design an eating regimen that will uphold muscle development, weight reduction, and generally wellbeing.

Bodybuilding is an activity that requires immense dedication and effort to achieve the desired results. It involves rigorous training, discipline, and a balanced diet to build muscle and strength. While bodybuilding has been traditionally associated with men, there has been a growing interest in women participating in this activity. However, women over the age of 40 may face unique challenges when it comes to bodybuilding, especially when it comes to their diet.

This book aims to provide a comprehensive guide for women over 40 who are interested in bodybuilding and want to optimize their diet to achieve their fitness goals. We will discuss the specific dietary requirements for women in this age group, including the right balance of macronutrients, vitamins, and minerals necessary for muscle growth and repair. We will also cover the best food sources to obtain these nutrients and how to incorporate them into a healthy diet plan.

Chapter One

1.1 Basics of bodybuilding

Dieting is an act of managing and controlling the intake of food determined to accomplish a specific wellbeing result, like weight reduction or further developed wellbeing. It includes making changes to one's dietary patterns and frequently includes following a particular eating regimen plan, for example, decreasing calorie consumption, restricting specific nutrition classes, or expanding protein admission.

Dieting is frequently attempted for weight reduction purposes, yet it can likewise be utilized to deal with specific ailments, like diabetes or coronary illness. In any case, it's vital to take note of that not all diets are sound or powerful, and outrageous or prohibitive eating regimens can prompt negative well being results.

Fruitful consuming less calories requires a mix of

good dieting propensities, standard activity, and a reasonable way to deal with food consumption.

1.2 Nutritional needs for women over 40

As ladies age, their wholesome necessities change. Here are a few significant supplements that ladies more than 40 ought to make a point to remember

for their weight control plans:
- Protein
- Carbohydrate
- Fats
- Vitamins
- Minerals

1.3 Importance of Protein, Carbohydrates, Fats, Vitamins and Minerals

1.3.1 Protein

Proteins are fundamental macronutrients that assume a significant part in a sound eating regimen. They are comprised of chains of amino acids, and our bodies use them to assemble and fix tissues, including muscle tissue.

With regards to eating fewer carbs, protein is frequently underscored on the grounds that it can assist you with feeling more full for longer time frames, which might assist with weight reduction endeavors. Eating an eating regimen that is higher in protein may likewise assist with protecting bulk while you are shedding pounds, which can be significant for by and large wellbeing.

Furthermore, consuming satisfactory measures of protein is significant for keeping up with legitimate physical process, as it is engaged with many physiological cycles, like catalyst creation, chemical guideline, and insusceptible framework capability.

Nonetheless, it is vital to take note that consuming inordinate measures of protein can likewise have negative wellbeing impacts, remembering possible pressure for the kidneys and liver. Consuming protein with some restraint as a component of a fair diet is suggested. The specific measure of protein that is suitable for an individual can shift contingent upon variables like age, sex, weight, and action level.Protein is a fundamental macronutrient that assumes a few significant parts in the body. For ladies north of 40, protein turns out to be significantly more basic, as it assists with tending to a portion of the progressions that happen with maturing. Here are a portion of the essential motivations behind why protein is significant in the eating regimen of ladies more than 40 who are counting calories:

- Keeping up muscle mass: As we age, we will more often than not lose muscle mass, which can prompt a diminishing in strength and versatility. Protein is fundamental for building and keeping up with muscle, which is the reason ladies north of 40 must consume sufficient protein to forestall muscle misfortune.

- Supporting digestion: Protein has a higher thermic impact than carbs or fats, implying that it takes more energy to process and use protein. This can assist with supporting digestion and consume more calories, which can be particularly significant for ladies north of 40 who might have a more slow digestion.

- Supporting bone health: Protein is fundamental for the arrangement and upkeep of bones. As ladies age, they become more defenseless to bone misfortune and osteoporosis, so it's critical to consume sufficient protein to help bone wellbeing.

- Diminishing craving: Protein is profoundly satisfying, and that implies that it can assist with lessening hunger and advance sensations of completion. One of the major advantages of getting enough protein is that it can reduce cravings and increase feelings of fullness, both of which can help with weight control.

1.3.2 Carbohydrates

Carbohydrates are a fundamental macronutrient that give energy to the body. They are tracked down in numerous food varieties, including grains, natural products, vegetables, and dairy items. With regards to consuming less calories, carbs can assume a critical part in deciding the outcome of the eating regimen.

Carbohydrates are frequently thought of "terrible" or "stuffing" by many individuals who are attempting to get more fit. Nonetheless, this isn't completely exact. Sugars are a significant wellspring of energy for the body, and an eating regimen that totally disposes of them can be hurtful to by and large wellbeing.

With regards to weight reduction, the key is to zero in on consuming the right kinds of starches. Complex carbs, like those tracked down in entire grains, natural products, and vegetables, are commonly more gainful than basic starches, like those tracked down in refined sugars and handled food varieties.

Food varieties high in complex starches give supported energy and assist with keeping you feeling full for longer time frames. They likewise will quite often be lower in calories than food varieties high in basic sugars. Consequently, picking complex carbs over basic starches can assist you with getting more fit and keep a solid eating regimen.

It's essential to take note of that everybody's dietary necessities are unique, and certain individuals might require more carbs than others relying upon their movement level, age, and by and large wellbeing. Talking with an enlisted dietitian or medical services proficient can assist you with deciding the perfect proportion of sugars to remember for your eating regimen. Here are a few justifications for why carbohydrates are significant in the eating regimen of ladies north of 40:

- Energy: Carbohydrates are the essential wellspring of energy for the body, and they give the energy expected to active work and day to day errands. This is particularly significant for ladies north of 40 who might have lower energy levels because of hormonal changes and different elements.

- Weight management: Carbohydrates are a significant part of a decent eating regimen, and they can assist ladies north of 40 with keeping a solid weight. Low-carbohydrates diets might bring about transient weight reduction, however they can be challenging to support over the long haul and may prompt supplement lacks.

• Fiber: Carbohydrates are a significant wellspring

of dietary fiber, which is fundamental for stomach related wellbeing and can assist with constipation, diverticulitis, and other digestive disorder. Ladies more than 40 might be at higher risk for these circumstances, making it particularly vital to consume sufficient measures of fiber.

- Supplements: Numerous carbohydrates rich food varieties are likewise great wellsprings of significant supplements, like nutrients, minerals, and cancer prevention agents. These supplements are significant for generally speaking wellbeing and can assist with forestalling age-related infections and conditions.

- Mood and Cognitive function: Carbohydrates can influence state of mind and mental capability by impacting the development of synapses in the cerebrum, like serotonin and dopamine. This is significant for ladies north of 40 who might be encountering hormonal changes that can influence state of mind and mental capability.

1.3.3 Fats

Fats are a fundamental supplement that assume a significant part in the eating routine of ladies north of 40. It is essential to take note of that not all fats are made equivalent. A few fats, for example, saturated and trans fats, can build the risk of heart attack and ought to be restricted in the eating routine. All things considered, ladies north of

40 ought to zero in on devouring healthy fats, for example, monounsaturated and polyunsaturated fats, which can be found in food varieties like nuts, seeds, avocados, greasy fish, and olive oil. Consuming fats with some restraint as a feature of a decent diet is likewise significant. Here are a few justifications for why fats are significant in

the eating routine of ladies north of 40:

- Brain function: Fats are significant for mind capability and can work on mental capability and memory. This is particularly significant for ladies north of 40 who might encounter mental degradation as they age.

- Hormone production: Fats are important for the development of hormones, including estrogen and progesterone, which are fundamental for ladies' conceptive wellbeing. As ladies north of 40 experience hormonal changes because of menopause, consuming satisfactory measures of sound fats can uphold chemical guidelines.

- Nutrient absorption: Fats assist the body with retaining fat-soluble nutrients, like nutrients A, D, E, and K, which are fundamental for generally speaking wellbeing.

- Energy: Fats are a wellspring of energy for

the body and can assist
ladies north of 40 with
keeping up with their
energy levels over the
course of the day.

• Skin health: Sound fats,
like omega-3 fatty acid,
can further develop skin
wellbeing by decreasing
inflammation and
further developing
hydration levels.

- Appetite control: Consuming sound fats can advance sensations of totality and assist with controlling hunger, which can be valuable for weight the board.

1.4 ROLE OF VITAMINS AND MINERALS

1.4.1 Vitamins

Women over 40 who want to keep their health and wellbeing should include vitamins in their diet. In the setting of dieting for women over 40, vitamins are crucial in the following ways:
Immune system: Vitamins A, C, and E, as well as vitamin D, are essential for immune system health.

Women's immune systems may deteriorate with age, making them more prone to infections and ailments. Getting enough of these micronutrients can support immune system health and shield you from disease.

- Bone health: Vitamins D and K are crucial for bone health because they facilitate calcium absorption and bone formation in the body. A sufficient intake of these vitamins can help keep bone health as women over 40 are more susceptible to osteoporosis and bone fractures.

- Heart health: Vitamins B6, B12, and folate are important for heart health, as they help lower homocysteine levels, a marker of cardiovascular disease risk. Consuming foods that are rich in these vitamins, such as leafy greens, nuts, and fortified cereals, can help promote heart health.

- Eye health: Vitamins A, C, and E have antioxidant properties that help safeguard the eyes from oxidative stress and age-related damage, making them crucial for eye health.

- Skin health: The antioxidant qualities of vitamins C and E, which help shield the skin from free radical damage, are crucial for maintaining healthy skin.

It's crucial to remember that eating a balanced, varied

diet that includes a range of nutrient-dense foods is the best way to make sure you're getting enough vitamins. Vitamin supplements may be required in some situations to resolve deficiencies, but it is always advised to speak with a healthcare provider before taking supplements. It's also essential to let your healthcare provider know about any supplements you're taking because some vitamins may interact with certain medications.

1.4.2 Minerals

Minerals are necessary nutrients that are crucial to many bodily physiological functions. In the context of dieting for women over 40, minerals can be essential in the following ways:

Bone health: Minerals like calcium, magnesium, and phosphate are crucial for healthy bones. The risk of osteoporosis is greater in women over 40, so getting enough of these minerals can help maintain bone density and lower the chance of fractures.

- Muscle function: Minerals like potassium, magnesium, and calcium are crucial for proper muscle performance. Consuming enough of these minerals can help keep muscle mass and strength in women as they age because they may experience muscle loss as they age.

- Heart health: Minerals like sodium, potassium, and magnesium are crucial for heart function. Blood pressure can rise as a result of eating too much sodium, which is a danger factor for heart disease. On the other hand, getting enough potassium and magnesium into your diet can help lower blood pressure and lower your chance of developing heart disease.

- Blood sugar: Magnesium and chromium are crucial nutrients for controlling blood sugar. Consuming enough of these minerals can help improve insulin sensitivity and control blood sugar levels because women over 40 may have a higher risk of getting type 2 diabetes.

- Hormone regulation: Minerals like iron, zinc, and selenium are crucial for hormone control. While zinc and selenium are crucial for endocrine and reproductive health, iron is crucial for the creation of red blood cells.

It's crucial to remember that eating a balanced, varied diet that includes a variety of nutrient-dense foods is the best way to guarantee sufficient mineral intake. Mineral supplements may be required in some circumstances to resolve deficiencies, but it is always advised to speak with a healthcare provider before taking supplements.

Chapter Two

2.1 Building Your Bodybuilding Diet Plan

2.1.1 Calculating Daily Caloric Need

Calories are a unit of measurement for food's energy content. A calorie is specifically the quantity of energy needed to increase the temperature of 1 gram of water by 1 degree Celsius. Typically, when discussing diet, we use the unit kilocalories (kcal), which stands for 1000 calories.

This is the standard measurement unit for food's energy level.When we consume, our bodies disassemble it into its constituent proteins, fats, and carbohydrates and use the energy released to power various physiological functions. A food's caloric content is determined by how much of each of these macronutrients it includes.

Every day, the body expends a certain amount of calories just to maintain essential processes like breathing and blood circulation. The basal metabolic rate (BMR), which changes with age, sex, body composition, and activity level, is referred to as this. When we consume more calories than our bodies require for these essential processes, the extra calories are stored as fat, which can eventually cause weight increase. On the other hand, when we eat fewer calories than our bodies require, the body turns to fat reserves for energy. Over time, this can result in weight loss. Thus, knowing how many calories are in the foods we eat and how many calories our bodies require can support overall health and help us keep a healthy weight. Understanding calories is crucial when dieting for women over 40 because it can support general health and aid in weight management. Women's metabolisms tend to slow down as they get older, so they need fewer calories than they did when they were younger to keep their weight and energy levels. A decline in metabolic rate can also be facilitated by hormonal changes and a loss of muscular mass. It's crucial for women over 40 to ingest the right number of calories based on their unique requirements if they want to maintain a healthy weight. Overeating can cause weight gain and raise one's chance of developing chronic conditions like diabetes, heart disease, and some types of cancer. Contrarily, eating insufficient calories can result in nutrient deficiencies and a loss of muscle mass.

The precise calorie requirement will change based on factors like age, sex, weight, height, and level of activity. Women over 40 should generally strive to eat a balanced and diverse diet that includes a range of nutrient-dense foods, such as fruits, vegetables, whole grains, lean proteins, and healthy fats. Additionally, it's critical to pay attention to serving sizes and restrict the intake of foods that are high in calories, fat, and sugar. In general, a healthy diet for women over 40 can include a knowledge of calories and how they relate to weight management.

The calculation of a woman's caloric needs after the age of 40 depends on a number of variables, including her age, height, weight, body composition, and degree of activity. Here are a few ways to calculate calorie requirements:

1.Basal Metabolic Rate (BMR) calculation: Calculating the basal metabolic rate (BMR) The BMR is the amount

of energy needed by the body at rest to sustain fundamental processes like breathing, circulation, and digestion. For estimating BMR in women, the Harris-Benedict equation is a frequently used formula:
BMR is calculated as 655 + 9.6 x weight in kg + 1.8 x height in

centimeters - (4.7 x age
in years)

Your daily caloric requirements can be determined by multiplying your BMR by an activity factor. The energy required for physical activity is taken into consideration by the activity factor, which ranges from 1.2 for sedentary lifestyles to 2.2 for extremely active lifestyles. For instance, if you have a moderate activity level (activity factor of 1.5) and your BMR is 1400 calories, your estimated daily caloric requirements are 2100 calories (1400 x 1.5).

The amount of physical activity a woman over the age of 40 engages in will determine the activity factor used in BMR calculations. In general, older women may be slightly less active than younger women, but this will vary depending on personal traits like occupation, hobbies, and degree of fitness.

For BMR calculations depending on activity level, consider the following general activity factors:

The amount of physical activity a woman over the age of 40 engages in will determine the activity factor used in BMR calculations.

In general, older women may be slightly less active than younger women, but this will vary depending on personal traits like occupation, hobbies, and degree of fitness.

For BMR calculations depending on activity level, consider the following general activity factors:

- Sedentary (little or no exercise, desk job): 1.2 - 1.3
- Lightly active (light exercise or sports 1-3 days a week): 1.4 - 1.5

- Moderately active (moderate exercise or sports 3-5 days a week): 1.6 - 1.7

- Very active (hard exercise or sports 6-7 days a week): 1.8 - 1.9

- Extremely active (very hard exercise or sports, physical job or training twice a day): 2.0 - 2.2

For instance, the activity factor for a woman over 40 with a BMR of 1400 calories and a fairly active lifestyle would be 1.6 to 1.7. 1400 multiplied by the activity component yields a daily caloric requirement of roughly 2240–2380 calories. It's essential to remember that these activity factors only offer broad estimates and might not accurately reflect each person's needs. A registered dietitian, for example, can help you determine the right caloric intake based on your needs and objectives by consulting with you. In order to promote general health, it's also crucial to follow a varied, balanced diet that includes a range of nutrient-rich foods.

2. Total Energy Expenditure (TEE) calculation: TEE considers both BMR and physical exercise, which might give a more precise estimation of daily calorie

requirements. TEE can be calculated online or using wearable fitness trackers that consider individual characteristics like age, sex, weight, height, and exercise level.

3.Body Composition analysis: Lean mass and fat mass in the body can be determined by measuring body composition, such as through dual-energy x-ray absorptiometry or bioelectrical impedance measurement. Based on each person's unique metabolic rates and activity levels, this information can then be used to determine a more precise estimate of their caloric requirements.

While these techniques can give a decent indication of caloric requirements, it's important to keep in mind that they might not be perfect and should only be used as a guide rather than a precise prescription. A registered dietitian, for example, can help you determine the right caloric intake based on your needs and objectives by consulting with you. In order to promote general health, it's also crucial to follow a varied, balanced diet that includes a range of nutrient-rich foods.

2.1.2 Determining Macronutrients Requirements

To provide energy and support a variety of bodily functions, the diet must contain macronutrients in relatively significant amounts. Macronutrients plays a role in weight management and overall health. Consuming an appropriate balance of macronutrients can help regulate appetite, improve body composition, and reduce the risk of chronic diseases such as heart disease and diabetes. By giving the body energy, supporting the development and maintenance of muscle and other tissues, and assisting in the maintenance of general health and wellbeing, macronutrients play a critical role in the diet of women over 40. The suggested macronutrient breakdown for ladies over 40 is, however, as a general rule:

- Carbohydrates: Aim for 45–65% of your daily calories to come from carbs for women over 40. The majority of this should consist of complex carbohydrates, like those found in whole grains, fruits, veggies, and legumes.

- Protein: Over-40 women should try to get 10 to 35 percent of their daily energy from protein. Among these sources are lean meats, seafood, poultry, dairy products, legumes, and nuts.

- Fat: Over-40-year-old women should strive to get 20 to 35 percent of their daily calories from healthy fats. These can come from foods like nuts, seeds, avocados, extra virgin olive oil, and fatty seafood.

Age, weight, height, activity level, and general health state are all individual considerations when determining the macronutrient requirements for women over 40. The following are some basic guidelines:

- Calculate daily calorie needs: Calories required for everyday maintenance should be calculated. An online calorie counter can be used to determine this, or a certified dietitian or healthcare provider can be consulted.

- Determine macronutrient

breakdown: Calculate the suggested macronutrient split for carbohydrates, proteins, and fats based on the daily caloric requirements. According to general guidelines, women over 40 should consume 45–65% of their calories from carbs, 10–35% from protein, and 20–35% from fats.

- Adjust macronutrient intake: Depending on personal circumstances, adjust your consumption of macronutrients. For instance, active women over 40 may need a larger proportion of carbohydrates and proteins to support their level of exercise and muscle maintenance. In contrast, older women

who are trying to lose
weight might need a
smaller proportion of
carbohydrates and fats
to do so.

- Monitor intake and
adjust as necessary:
Intake of macronutrients
should be monitored and
modified as required
based on each person's
needs and goals. Making
adjustments and

developing a personalized nutrition plan can benefit from speaking with a healthcare expert or registered dietitian.

2.2 Sample Meal Plans And Recipes

Sample Meal Plans

Meal planning is an effective instrument for

sustaining a healthy diet and way of life and can support women over 40 in achieving their wellness and health objectives. Just like every other thing, with proper knowledge meal planning can be used to acquire desired results, if carefully orchestrated, a bodybuilding diet should be created for women over 40 that supports muscle development and recovery while also enhancing general health and wellbeing.

Here are few reasons why:

a. Meal planning can be a useful weight management aid for women over 40 who may have difficulty losing weight due to changes in metabolism, hormones, and lifestyle factors. We can manage portion sizes, prevent overeating, and make sure we are ingesting the proper ratio of macronutrients to support weight loss or maintenance by planning our meals and snacks.

b.It saves time and money: By preplanning your meals, you can save time and money by cooking in bulk, doing your grocery buying in bulk, and avoiding food waste. Having a plan for what you're going to consume ahead of time can help you stay on track with your healthy eating habits by reducing stress and decision fatigue.

c.By lowering stress and decision fatigue, making a plan for your meals in advance can help you stay on task with your healthy eating habits.

d.Planning your meals can assist you in portion control, which can help you avoid overeating and encourage improved digestion.

e.Aids in ensuring sufficient nutrient intake: As we age, our nutritional requirements change, making it harder to get all the nutrients we require from our diets. We can make sure we are getting a variety of nutrient-dense foods and meeting our unique nutrient requirements by pre-planning our meals.

f. Provides variety: By organizing your meals in preparation, you can include a variety of foods and flavors in your diet, preventing mealtime boredom.

g.It reduces food waste: Planning your meals in advance allows you to purchase only the ingredients you actually need, minimizing food waste.

h.It can be simpler to make healthy decisions throughout the day when we have planned and easily available healthy meals and snacks. When we are busy or stressed, this can help us prevent impulsive eating or choosing less healthy choices.

An example menu is provided below:

Meal one (1)

1 sliced banana, 1 spoonful of almond butter, and 1 cup of oatmeal
a single scrambled egg and two Fegg yolks
one coffee or tea cup

Meal Two (2)

One whey protein shake prepared with one scoop, one cup of almond milk, and half a cup of frozen berries.

Meal Three (3)

Chicken breast, broiled, weighing 4 ounces
1 cup of rice

a single cup of grilled veggies (such as broccoli, cauliflower, and carrots)

Meal Four (4)

1 apple
1 ounce of almonds or walnuts

Meal Five (5)

4 ounces of fish, grilled
1 sweet potato

1 cup of green beans, cooked

Meal Six (6)

1/2 cup of mixed berries, 1 spoonful of honey, and 1 cup of Greek yogurt

In order to support muscle growth and recovery, this meal plan offers a balance of carbohydrates, proteins, and healthy fats. It also includes necessary vitamins and minerals to support general health. It's crucial to modify the macronutrient distribution and portion sizes according to each person's requirements and goals. Making a custom meal plan may benefit from advice from a registered dietitian or healthcare expert. For muscle function and recovery, it's also crucial to remain hydrated throughout the day by drinking lots of water.

MEAL PLAN One (1)

1 cup of oatmeal: Carbohydrates, which give your body energy and promote muscle growth, are found in abundance in oatmeal. Additionally, it has fiber, which aids in metabolism and makes you feel fuller for longer. In

order to avoid added sugars and artificial tastes, choose basic, unsweetened oatmeal. One tablespoon of almond butter contains healthy fats that are vital for the creation of hormones and brain activity. Protein, which is necessary for both muscle development and repair, is also present.

One cut banana The nutrients potassium, vitamin C, and carbs are all abundant in bananas. Potassium aids in maintaining the body's fluid equilibrium, and vitamin C promotes immune health.

2 egg yolks and 1 scrambled egg: Protein, which is necessary for muscle development and repair, is found in abundance in eggs. Additionally, important nutrients like choline and vitamin D are found in egg yolks. Egg whites can aid in

reducing total calorie and fat intake.

1 cup of coffee or tea: Caffeine, which is present in coffee and tea, can help improve concentration and energy levels during exercise. To prevent sleep disruption, it's crucial to keep caffeine consumption to a minimum and to avoid consuming it too close to bedtime.

Meal Plan Two (2)

1 whey protein shake with 1 cup of almond milk, 1 scoop of the protein, and 1/2 cup of frozen berries: Having a quick supply of protein and carbohydrates in between meals or after exercise is simple and convenient with this protein shake. Whey protein is the best type of protein for muscle development and recovery

because it digests quickly and is quickly absorbed by the body. In addition to providing antioxidants and vitamins, almond milk is a low-calorie, dairy-free substitute for regular milk. Frozen berries also do the same.

One scoop of whey protein is a high-quality protein source that the body can readily digest. It has every important amino acid that the body requires to maintain and grow muscle. Almond milk contains calcium, vitamin D, and vitamin E in moderate amounts per cup. Additionally, it has few calories and no cholesterol or fatty fat.

Frozen berries, 1/2 cup: Berries are an excellent source of vitamins, fiber, and antioxidants. They can flavor and sweeten the protein drink and are also low in calories. Strawberries, blueberries, raspberries, and blackberries are a few tasty berry choices.

Meal Three (3)

4 ounces of grilled chicken breast: Lean protein is essential for muscle development and healing and is abundant in chicken

breast. It is a healthy option for those monitoring their calorie intake because it is low in fat and calories.

Cooked sweet potatoes in 1 cup: The body gets its energy from complex carbohydrates, which sweet potatoes are an excellent source of. Additionally, they contain fiber, vitamins, and minerals like manganese, potassium, and vitamin A.

Steamed broccoli, 1 cup: Broccoli is an excellent source of fiber, potassium, vitamin C, and other vitamins and minerals. It is a healthy option for those watching their calorie consumption because it is also low in calories.

1 tablespoon of olive oil: Monounsaturated fats, which are found in olive oil and are healthy, can help lower cholesterol and lower

the chance of heart disease. Additionally, it is an excellent source of vitamin E, an antioxidant that aids in defending the body's cells against harm.

Meal Four (4)

1 apple: Apples are an excellent source of antioxidants, fiber, and vitamins. They are a calorie-efficient snack

choice due to their low calorie content.

2 teaspoons of almond butter: Almond butter is an excellent source of protein, fiber, and good fats. Magnesium, calcium, and vitamin E are all abundant in it.

1 rice cake: A low-calorie and low-fat snack choice is rice cakes. They also contain plenty of carbs,

which the body can use as fuel.

Cinnamon: This snack benefits from the flavorful and nutritious inclusion of cinnamon. It has been demonstrated to have anti-inflammatory effects, and it might also assist in controlling blood sugar levels.

Meal Five (5)

Salmon is a good source of lean protein and omega-3 fatty acids, which can help to reduce inflammation and improve heart health. 4 ounces of grilled salmon are a good example of this. Additionally, it is an excellent source of vitamin D, which is crucial for strong bones.

One cup of quinoa contains both complex carbs and

protein in reasonable amounts. Additionally, it is an excellent source of fiber, vitamins, and minerals like iron and magnesium.

Steamed asparagus in a cup: Fiber, vitamins, and minerals like vitamin K, vitamin C, and folate are all present in asparagus in adequate amounts. It is a healthy option for those watching their calorie consumption because it is also low in calories.

Balsamic vinegar, 1 tablespoon: Balsamic vinegar is a flavorful and beneficial ingredient to this dish. It has few calories and can make dishes taste better without adding more salt or fat.

Meal six (6)

1 scoop of whey protein powder: For athletes and bodybuilders, whey protein powder is a well-liked and practical supply of protein. It can promote muscle growth and recovery and is readily absorbed by the body.

Unsweetened almond milk is a low-calorie and low-fat substitute for dairy milk, making one cup of it ideal. Additionally, it is an excellent source of vitamin D, calcium, and E.

A decent source of fiber, protein, and good fats is one tablespoon of chia seeds. Additionally, they contain plenty of omega-3 fatty acids, which can help to lower inflammation and enhance cardiac health.

One teaspoon of honey can enhance the flavor of food without adding extra sugar or artificial sweeteners.

Honey is a natural sweetener.

Recipes

Meal One (1)

Egg White and Vegetable Omelette

Ingredients:

3 white egg yolks

veggies, chopped into a half-cup (such as spinach, bell peppers, onions, and mushrooms)
Olive oil, 1 drop
pepper and salt as desired

Instructions:

Olive oil is added to a non-stick pan that is already hot.

Add the chopped veggies to the skillet and cook them until they are soft.
Beat the egg whites in a small dish The olive oil should be heated over medium heat in a different pan.
until they are foamy.
Over the veggies in the skillet, pour the egg whites.
Till the bottom is firm, cook the omelette for 2 to 3 minutes.

The omelet should be folded in half with a spatula and cooked for an additional minute, or until the egg whites are completely done. Add pepper and salt to suit.

Meal Two (2)

Roasted Chicken and Veggies

Ingredients:

grilled chicken breast weighing 4 lbs.
one cup of various veggies (such as zucchini, bell peppers, onions, and broccoli)
Olive oil, 1 teaspoonful
pepper and salt as desired

Instructions:

Grill or grill skillet should be heated to medium-high.

Add salt and pepper to the poultry breast before cooking.

The chicken breast should be roasted through, about 5-7 minutes per side, on the grill.

The olive oil should be heated over medium heat in a different pan.

The mixed veggies should be added to the skillet and

cooked for 3–4 minutes, or until tender.

Add salt and pepper to taste and season the veggies.

The sautéed veggies should be served alongside the grilled chicken breast.

Meal Three (3)

Avocado-Tuna Salad with Mixed Vegetables

Ingredients:

3 ounces of drained canned salmon
1/2 avocado, diced
1 cup of leaves, various (such as spinach, arugula, and kale)
Olive oil, 1 teaspoonful
Balsamic vinegar, 1 teaspoonful
pepper and salt as desired

Instructions

Avocado dice and canned tuna should be combined in a dish.

To prepare the dressing, combine the olive oil, balsamic vinegar, salt, and pepper in a different bowl.

In the dish with the tuna and avocado, add the mixed greens.

The lettuce should be tossed after the dressing has been added.

Meal Four (4)

Roasted vegetables and baked salmon

Ingredients:

4 ounces of broiled salmon fillet
1 cup of roasted veggies, mixed (such as asparagus,

cherry tomatoes, and Brussels sprouts)
Olive oil, 1 teaspoonful
pepper and salt as desired

Instructions

Turn the oven on to 375°F.
With salt and pepper, season the salmon piece.
On a baking tray covered with parchment paper, put the salmon fillet.

Salmon piece should be baked for 15 to 20 minutes, or until done.

Mix the veggies in a separate baking dish and toss with the olive oil, salt, and pepper.

The veggies should be baked for 15 to 20 minutes, or until tender.

Along with the baked salmon fillet, serve roasted veggies.

Meal Five (5)

Sweet potato and broccoli with grilled chicken

Ingredients:

grilled chicken breast weighing 4 lbs.
1 diced tiny sweet potato
one cup of broccoli stems
Olive oil, 1 teaspoonful
pepper and salt as desired

Instructions

Grill or grill skillet should be heated to medium-high. Sprinkle salt and pepper on the chicken breast.

The chicken breast should be cooked through after 6-7 minutes on each side of the grill.

Sliced sweet potatoes should be cooked in olive oil over medium heat until they are soft.

In a different pot, steam the broccoli florets for 3 to 5 minutes, or until they are vibrant green and soft. Serve the grilled chicken breast with the sweet potato and broccoli on the side.

Meal Six (6)

Roasted salmon with quinoa and asparagus

Ingredients:

4 ounces of grilled fish
 1 cup cooked rice
a single cup of asparagus stalks
Olive oil, 1 teaspoonful
pepper and salt as desired

Instructions

Grill or grill skillet should be heated to medium-high.

Add salt and pepper to the fish to season it.

The salmon should be roasted through on the grill for 5 to 6 minutes on each side.

The asparagus stalks should be cooked in olive oil over medium heat until they are tender and just beginning to char.

As directed on the box, prepare the quinoa.

The Package instructions

To get rid of any bitterness, rinse the quinoa under running water in about fine-mesh colander.

The quinoa should be combined with water or veggie broth in a medium saucepan. Adding a dash of salt is optional.

Over high heat, bring the liquid to a boil.

When the water has boiled, turn the heat down to medium and put a lid on the pot.

Until the water has been drained and the quinoa is tender, simmer the quinoa for 15 to 20 minutes.

After turning off the heat, leave the pot covered for five minutes.

Serve the prepared quinoa and asparagus alongside the grilled salmon.

Note: Feel free to change portion sizes in this recipe to fit your tastes. When preparing meals, it's crucial to take your unique dietary requirements and objectives into account.

Chapter Three

3.1 Meal Timing

The term "meal timing" refers to the habit of consuming meals and snacks at regular intervals throughout the day, usually separated by 3–4 hours. This can lower blood sugar levels, discourage overeating, and encourage sound metabolism. Women over 40 are generally advised to eat three main meals per day, with 1-2 snacks in between as required. Depending on personal preferences and lifestyle factors, the timing of these meals and snacks may vary, but it's essential to avoid skipping meals or going for extended periods without eating because doing so can cause overeating or bingeing in the future.

Women over 40 are generally advised to eat three main meals per day, with 1-2 snacks in between as required. Depending on personal preferences and lifestyle factors, the timing of these meals and snacks may vary, but it's essential to avoid skipping meals or going for extended periods without eating because doing so can cause overeating or bingeing in the future.

Meal timing is important when dieting for a variety of reasons, including:

1. Regulating Blood Sugar Levels: regulating blood sugar levels is an important health benefit of properly timing meals. Blood sugar, also known as glucose, is the primary source of energy for the body's cells. However, too much glucose in the bloodstream can be harmful and lead to a condition known as

hyperglycemia. Our blood sugar levels can quickly rise after eating a meal, particularly one that is rich in carbohydrates. A rise in insulin, a hormone that helps control blood sugar levels by transporting glucose from the circulation into the cells for energy, may result from this. The body can develop insulin resistance if insulin levels are kept elevated for an extended period of time, which can result in a number of health issues, including type 2 diabetes, heart disease, and obesity. Meals and snacks should be timed appropriately to help avoid these blood sugar surges and crashes. For instance, consuming a balanced meal rich in protein, good fats, and complex carbohydrates can aid in reducing the rate at which glucose is absorbed into the bloodstream, causing blood sugar levels to increase more gradually. Regular meal times throughout the day can also aid in keeping blood sugar levels steady, avoiding dips that might otherwise result in fatigue, wooziness, and cravings for unhealthy foods. Women over 40 can promote overall health and wellness while also avoiding the onset of chronic health conditions like type 2 diabetes and heart disease by controlling blood sugar levels through appropriate meal timing.

2. Avoid Skipping Meals: Going without food for extended stretches of time or skipping meals can cause overeating or poor food decisions because of extreme hunger. Ultimately, this can undermine weight loss attempts and result in blood sugar

imbalances, which can have an impact on one's energy levels and general health. Your body enters a "starvation state" when you skip meals, which causes it to slow down metabolism in order to preserve energy. As a consequence, the body starts utilizing muscle tissue as fuel rather than fat. For women over 40 who are at risk of losing muscle mass as a result of hormonal changes, this muscle loss can reduce total strength. In addition, missing meals may cause binge eating later in the day or the intake of unhealthy snacks as a means of satisfying hunger. Regular meals and snacks help maintain steady blood sugar levels and constant energy levels throughout the day. Better food options and a greater likelihood of fulfilling nutrient requirements can result from this, which will eventually support weight loss and general health.

3. Supporting Healthy Digestion: Your body learns to anticipate the

arrival of food and your digestive system gets ready for it when you consume your meals at the same time every day. Better digestion and nutrient absorption from your diet may result from this. Additionally, timing your meals correctly can help you prevent digestive discomforts like indigestion and bloating that can happen when you consume too much or too little at once. For instance, your body might not have enough time to properly digest a big meal if you consume it late at night and then go to bed right away. This may result in bloating, indigestion, and other stomach problems. Your body, however, has an easier time digesting and absorbing the nutrients from your food if you consume smaller, more frequent meals throughout the day. In conclusion, eating at the right times of day can help your digestion and ensure that your body gets all the nutrition it needs from food.

4.Boosting Metabolism: Another significant advantage of scheduling your meals correctly is that it can increase metabolism. Your body uses the metabolic process to transform sustenance into usable energy. Your body expends calories while you consume in order to digest and assimilate the nutrients from the food.

Thermic impact of food is what's responsible for this (TEF). The TEF can contribute up to 10% of your daily caloric burn and is greatest in the few hours following a meal. You can increase your metabolism and maximize the TEF by timing your meals correctly. As your body is continuously working to digest and absorb nutrients, eating smaller, more frequent meals throughout the day can help keep your metabolism elevated. This is why eating 5–6 small meals per day, as opposed to 2-3 big ones, is advised by many nutritionists. Eating your largest meal of the day early in the day may also help increase metabolism, according to some studies. According to one study, individuals who ate a high-calorie breakfast and a low-calorie dinner lost more weight and had lower levels of body fat than people who did the opposite. Overall, eating at the right times can help you maximize your metabolism, enhance your body's capacity to expend calories, and help you shed pounds.

5. Promoting healthy weight management: The timing of your meals can also help older women control their weight in a healthy way. This is due to the fact that it aids in appetite control and discourages binge eating, which can result

in weight gain. Evenly spaced meals can aid in preventing hunger and lessen the likelihood that unhealthy snacks will be consumed throughout the day. The blood sugar levels can be kept stable by eating smaller, more frequent meals. This can help to avoid spikes and crashes that can cause cravings and overeating. A further strategy for weight management is to consume a bigger meal earlier in the day and a smaller meal later in the day. This is due to the fact that the body's metabolism tends to be greater in the morning and slower in the evening. A larger meal early in the day can give you the energy you need for work and exercise, while a smaller meal later in the day can help you avoid overeating and sleep better. It's important to remember that while meal timing can be a useful tool for managing weight, for best results, it should be used in conjunction with a balanced and nutritious diet, consistent exercise, and enough rest.

6. Providing sustained energy: The scheduling of meals can also be very important for sustaining energy levels throughout the day. Eat meals and refreshments at regular intervals throughout the day to maintain blood sugar levels and avoid energy slumps. This is crucial for women over 40 because their hormone

levels may fluctuate and have an impact on their energy levels. You may experience fatigue and sluggishness as a result of skipping meals or going too long between meals. On the other hand, ingesting a lot of food at once or right before bed can prevent you from falling asleep and make you feel groggy the next day.

You can make sure that your body has a steady amount of fuel to keep you energized throughout the day by properly timing and spacing out your meals and snacks. You'll be more able to stay focused and productive as a result, as well as adhere to your exercise and nutrition plan.

For ladies over 40 who want to optimize their diet and reach their health and fitness objectives, the following might be a suggested meal timing and spacing template:

- Following an hour of getting up, have breakfast.

- A mid-morning treat (2-3 hours after breakfast)

- 3–4 hours after the mid-morning nibble, lunch.

- Snack in the afternoon (2–3 hours after lunch).
- 3–4 hours after the midday snack, have dinner.

3.2 Portion Control

A dietary strategy known as portion control entails limiting the amount of food and calories eaten at meals and snacks. It involves consuming just enough food to satisfy one's nutritional requirements without going overboard, which can result in weight gain and other health issues. Instead of limiting particular foods or nutrients, portion control concentrates on limiting the amount of food consumed. Portion control can be especially helpful for women over 40 because as metabolism gradually slows down with age, it becomes easier to put on weight. Women who control their portions can keep a healthy weight, control their blood sugar levels, and lower their risk of developing chronic illnesses like diabetes and heart disease. When it comes to dieting for women over 40, there are a number of successful portion control techniques. Here are a few examples:

1. Use Smaller Plates: A quick and easy way for ladies over 40 to control their portion sizes when dieting is to use smaller plates. With a smaller

plate, individuals are more likely to serve themselves smaller servings, which results in fewer calories being consumed. According to research, when offered a larger plate, people prefer to serve themselves larger portions, which can result in overeating and weight gain. By giving the impression that the plate is full even though the portion size is smaller, using a smaller plate can help avoid this. It's crucial to pick a plate that is the right size if you want to use smaller plates successfully for portion control. A plate that is too big might make portion control impossible while a plate that is too tiny might not have enough food to sate hunger. The diameter of a typical dinner dish shouldn't exceed 10 inches, while the diameter of a salad plate shouldn't exceed 7 inches. When putting food on a platter, try to cover half of it with non-starchy vegetables, one-fourth of it with lean protein, and one-fourth of it with complex carbohydrates. It is crucial to eat slowly and mindfully, savoring each mouthful, and paying attention to feelings of fullness in addition to using smaller plates. This can aid in improved digestion and the reduction of overeating.

2.Measure Your Food: Using measuring

implements, such as spoons, measuring cups, and food scales, to precisely measure out food is another efficient portion control technique. This makes it possible to precisely monitor the amount of food consumed and can lessen the risk of overeating. When it comes to calorie-dense foods like nuts, oils, and dressings, which can rapidly build up in terms of calories if portions are not controlled, using measuring tools can be especially helpful. Furthermore, it's crucial to keep in mind that portion control does not necessarily entail limiting oneself to tiny servings or avoiding particular foods entirely. Finding a balance and being aware of how much is ingested are key. Utilizing measuring devices allows people to consume their favored foods in moderation without feeling deprived or overindulging.

3. Use Visual Cues: The technique of using visual cues for portion control includes making comparisons and using

familiar items to help determine the right portion sizes. For those who struggle to weigh or measure their meals, this method may be helpful. Visual Cues for portion control can be seen in the following instances:

- Using your hand: Using your hand can be a simple and

effective way to gauge portion amounts. A serving of protein, for instance, is roughly the size of your hand, whereas a serving of fats or oils is roughly the size of your thumb.

- Using familiar items as reference points is another method of using visual cues. A portion of cheese, for instance, can be compared to the size of four stacked dice, whereas a dish of cooked rice or pasta can be compared to the size of a tennis ball.

- Using the plate technique entails setting aside

portions of your plate for various dietary groups, such as half for vegetables, a quarter for protein, and a quarter for whole grains or starches. This can guarantee nutrient-dense meals and amounts that are balanced.

It is crucial to remember that visual signals for portion control are only approximations and might not be accurate. However, they can be a useful aid for promoting healthier eating habits and better comprehending appropriate portion sizes.

4.Avoid Distractions: A good portion control strategy is to avoid interruptions while eating. You can lose focus on your food consumption and overeat as a result of distractions like watching TV, using a phone, or reading. You become more conscious of what and how much you are eating when you consume without interruptions. You can stop consuming when you're satisfied because your body is more adept at detecting the signs of fullness. Additionally, eating carefully and with awareness can enhance digestion and increase food enjoyment.

Make a deliberate effort to turn off the TV, put your phone away, and sit at a table when you're eating to reduce distractions. Pay attention to what you're eating, chew methodically, and enjoy the flavors. This can increase your sense of fullness after eating and lessen the desire to overdo.

5. Eat Slowly: A straightforward but efficient way of portion control is eating slowly. Because our body

doesn't have enough time to recognize fullness when we consume too quickly, we frequently overeat. This may result in us consuming more calories than we need, which over time may cause us to acquire weight. We can savor our food, chew it fully, and appreciate eating when we consume slowly. Try to take smaller bites and chew each one completely before swallowing to practice eating leisurely. To savor your food more slowly, put your utensil down in between bites. You may be able to consume with greater satisfaction and enjoyment if you are more mindful and present while doing so.

According to research, eating more slowly can help you consume fewer calories, feel fuller, and lessen hunger. According to one research, eating slowly reduced calorie intake by 10% and increased feelings of fullness compared to eating rapidly. As a result, slowing down your eating can be a useful technique for managing your portions and weight.

6. Planning your meals is a good way to manage your portions because it gives your eating habits structure and control, which helps to avoid overeating. By making a plan, you can make sure that you are eating the correct amount of food

to satisfy your hunger without going over your calorie allotment. You can start by making a weekly meal plan that includes breakfast, lunch, supper, and snacks in order to portion-control your meals. This can assist you in making better decisions and lessen your desire to eat unhealthily.

Consider including lean protein, complex carbohydrates, healthy fats, as well as a range of fruits and veggies, when planning your meals. To make sure you are eating the right quantity of food, you can use portion control tools like measuring cups.

Additionally, avoid skipping meals or

dining on the go because these behaviors can result in overeating and unhealthy food selections. You can feel more satisfied and avoid overeating if you plan your meals in preparation and take the time to settle down and enjoy your meal.

7.	Practice Mindful Eating: Another useful

technique for portion management when it comes to dieting for women over 40 is mindful eating. The art of mindful eating involves eating while paying attention to the present instant without passing judgment. By doing so, you can become more conscious of your hunger and fullness cues and avoid overeating.

To help you practice conscious eating, here are some tips:

- Take your time and chew your food thoroughly.

- Pay attention to the food's flavor,

texture, and fragrance.

- Eat without any interruptions, such as using your phone or viewing TV.

- Eat slowly, chewing each mouthful completely.

- Take a moment between bites to

assess how hungry
or satiated you are.

- When you are
comfortably full
rather than stuffed,
cease eating. Pay
attention to your
body.

- Be careful not to
consume when
you're stressed or
bored.

3.3 Meal Frequency

The quantity of meals and refreshments a person eats each day is referred to as meal frequency. It is a part of the dietary pattern and has an impact on metabolic health as well as the general energy balance. Meal frequency is a term that varies depending on a person's culture and personal preferences, but is usually used to describe how many times they eat in a day. It can be as little as one meal per day (like intermittent fasting) or as many as six smaller meals spread out throughout the day. The quantity and scheduling of meals can affect other physiological processes like blood sugar control, satiety, and hunger. Nutritional studies on meal frequency, or the number of meals eaten each day, are still in progress. While there isn't a single best meal frequency for dieting women over 40, there are a number of possible health advantages to take into account

Metabolism And Weight Management: The process by which the body transforms food into energy that can be used for different processes, such as movement, digestion, and circulation, is known as metabolism. The metabolic rate is the amount of calories burned by the organism each day to maintain these processes. For some people, especially women over 40 who may experience a natural decline in metabolic rate as they age, eating frequently and in smaller amounts may help boost metabolism and assist in weight management. The body can remain in a constant condition of digestion by eating frequent, smaller meals, which may help increase the metabolic rate. Additionally, having small, frequent meals may help avoid overeating, which can result in weight gain, at later meals. By eating smaller, more frequent meals, individuals may be able to better control their calorie intake and avoid the overeating that can occur when meals are skipped or delayed.

It is significant to note that the complex connection between meal frequency and metabolism may differ depending on a person's age, gender, weight, and level of physical exercise. According to some studies, eating frequently and in small amounts may not have a major effect on everyone's metabolic rate and that other elements, such as diet quality and total calorie intake, may be more crucial for maintaining a healthy weight. As a result, while consuming frequently and in small amounts may be advantageous for some people, it is not a surefire way to lose weight and should only be used as one component of an overall healthy diet and way of life.

1.Blood Sugar Control: When it comes to dieting, blood sugar control is a crucial aspect to take into account, particularly for women over 40. Age-related declines in blood sugar regulation capacity can result in a number of health problems, such as insulin resistance, type 2 diabetes, and weight increase. Instead of having a few large meals throughout the day, eating several smaller meals frequently can help control blood sugar levels. This is because our systems release insulin after a meal to help control our blood sugar levels. Our bodies release a lot of insulin after a big meal, which can cause our blood sugar levels to fall dangerously low and leave us feeling weak and hungry. By maintaining more consistent blood sugar levels throughout the day, eating more frequent, smaller meals can help us prevent this problem.

Additionally, making the correct food choices can aid in blood sugar regulation. The glycemic index (GI), which gauges how fast a food raises blood sugar levels, should be considered when making food selections. White bread, pasta, and sugary snacks are examples of foods with a high GI that can cause blood sugar levels to rise and then crash, resulting in hunger and cravings. Choosing foods with a low GI, such as whole grains, fruits, veggies, and lean proteins, on the other hand, can help to stabilize blood sugar levels and lessen cravings and hunger. Women over 40 can help regulate their blood sugar levels and enhance their general health and wellbeing by eating frequently, in smaller amounts, and with low-GI foods.

2.Hunger And Satiety: When it comes to meal

frequency and dieting for women over 40, hunger and satiety are significant variables to take into account. In contrast to satiety, which is the feeling of fullness and pleasure experienced after eating, hunger is the discomfort or feeling of emptiness in the stomach that prompts the body to seek food. Hunger and satiety levels can be influenced by the regularity of meals. Eating more frequently—five or six short meals a day, for example—can aid in controlling hunger and preventing overeating. This is due to the fact that eating frequently can support stable blood sugar levels, which can aid in lowering cravings and appetite.

In contrast, having fewer, larger meals may result in greater blood sugar fluctuations, which may result in hunger and cravings. Additionally, eating bigger meals can stretch the stomach, making it harder to feel satisfied and filled. Managing hunger and satiety levels can be particularly crucial for dieting ladies over 40. Our metabolism slows down as we get older, which can make weight loss more challenging. Eating more frequently and in smaller portions can support weight reduction by maintaining a steady metabolism. Women may also experience changes in their hormonal balance as they mature, which may have an impact on their levels of satiety and hunger. For instance, due to changes in estrogen levels during menopause, appetite and cravings may rise. In order to control these changes in appetite and avoid overeating, consume more frequently and in smaller portions. Finding a meal frequency that suits your health and lifestyle is crucial when it comes to dieting for women over 40 and meal frequency. While other women might prefer larger, less frequent meals, some women may find that having smaller, more frequent meals helps control hunger and supports weight loss. Experimenting with various meal frequencies and paying attention to hunger and satiety levels can help determine what works best for you.

3.Nutrient Absorption: When we eat, our body transforms the food into vitamins, minerals, and nutrients like carbohydrates, proteins, and fats. These nutrients are then transported to various parts of the body where they are used for various purposes after being absorbed through the small intestine's lining. Eating more frequently can improve nutrient absorption by supplying the body with a steady stream of minerals all throughout the day. This is due to the fact that the body can only assimilate so many nutrients at once. The body may not be able to absorb all of the nutrients effectively if we consume larger, less frequent meals, resulting in nutrients that are wasted and pass through the body unutilized. Additionally, for optimum absorption, some nutrients, like calcium and iron, call for particular circumstances. For instance, calcium absorbs better when combined with other minerals like magnesium and vitamin D. More chances to eat these nutrient combinations can be obtained by eating smaller, more frequent meals, which may enhance absorption. Nutrient absorption is crucial for dieting women over 40 because the body may need extra nutrients to support good aging and fend off age-related illnesses. The body can get the nutrients it requires for optimum health by eating smaller, more frequent meals. It's crucial to remember that nutrient absorption is influenced by a variety of factors in addition to meal regularity. For optimum nutrient absorption and general health, eating a balanced diet that consists of a range of nutrient-dense foods, such as fruits, vegetables, whole grains, lean proteins, and healthy fats, is also crucial.

4. Energy Levels: For general health and wellbeing, it's crucial to maintain energy levels throughout the day. This is particularly true for women over 40, whose hormones may be changing and may have an impact on their energy levels. Meal

frequency can have a significant effect on energy levels when dieting. Small, frequent meals can help maintain blood sugar levels and avoid energy slumps throughout the day. Fatigue, weakness, and anger can occur when blood sugar levels fall too low. Women over 40 can prevent these energy crashes and keep a constant flow of energy throughout the day by eating smaller meals more frequently.

5. Regular mealtimes can also aid in reducing desires and overeating. People who miss meals or go too long without eating frequently experience excessive hunger and are therefore more likely to overeat or

choose unhealthy foods. Women over 40 can avoid this issue and maintain a more balanced and controlled approach to their diet by consuming smaller meals throughout the day. It's essential to remember, though, that eating frequently does not automatically result in long-lasting energy levels. The standard of the cuisine eaten is also very important. Choose meals that are high in nutrients and offer a steady supply of energy, such as whole grains, lean proteins, and healthy fats. Additionally, maintaining energy levels can be achieved by consuming plenty of water, avoiding caffeine, and abstaining from alcohol. In conclusion, women over 40 can keep sustained energy levels throughout the day while dieting by eating frequent, balanced meals. Women can optimize the advantages of frequent meals by making nutrient-dense food choices and maintaining hydration while maintaining their general health and wellbeing.

3.4 Making Healthy Food Choices While Eating Out Or Traveling

While traveling or dining out, it can be difficult to make healthy food decisions, but there are a number of tactics that women over 40 can use to do so:

1. Plan Ahead: If at all feasible, look up restaurants or food options in advance and select locations that provide healthier options. Choose places with menus that include fresh produce, lean protein, and whole

grains. Utilize the nutritional information that many eateries now include on their menus when choosing your meal.

2.Choose Wisely: When purchasing, go for dishes that have been grilled, baked, or steamed rather than those that have been cooked or sautéed.

Vinaigrettes or other light salad condiments should be used instead of creamy sauces. Avoid fatty cuts of meat and choose lean proteins like poultry or seafood. Request additional vegetables in lieu of starchy sides like fries or mashed potatoes.

3.Portion Control: Consider splitting a dish

with a companion or taking half of it home since restaurant portions are frequently much larger than required. When the food is delivered, ask for a to-go container, and fill it only halfway before you begin to consume.

4.Stay Hydrated: Drinking plenty of water is essential for overall health and can help you feel fuller, so take a reusable water bottle with you when traveling or going out.

5. Snack Smart: Bring wholesome snacks like whole-grain crackers, fresh produce, and nuts with you when you travel. By doing this, you can avoid getting too famished and

selecting unhealthy foods.

6. Don't Skip Meals: Avoid skipping meals whenever feasible because doing so can result in overeating or making unhealthy food choices.

7. Be Mindful: Finally, be mindful of your eating habits and pay attention

to how much you are consuming and how you feel. As you consume, take your time and savor each bite.

8. By using these strategies, you can make healthier food decisions while traveling or going out, and keep their overall health and wellbeing.

Chapter Four

4.0   Supplements   For Women Over 40

The purpose of supplements is to provide additional nutrients that may be lacking or insufficient in a person's regular diet. Supplements are dietary products. Supplements may be used in dieting for women over 40 to support general health and well-being as well as to address particular health issues that may be more prevalent in this age group. While some people may benefit from supplements, it's essential to remember that a balanced diet should always come first. The majority of the nutrients that the body requires can be obtained from a well-balanced, varied diet that includes a lot of fruits, veggies, whole grains, lean protein sources, and healthy fats.

However, some women over 40 might have particular nutrient requirements that cannot be satisfied by food alone. Women in this age group, for instance, may be more susceptible to osteoporosis and may profit from calcium and vitamin D supplements. Supplements containing omega-3 fatty acids may be beneficial for women over 40 because they may be at an increased risk of developing cardiac disease.

Probiotics, which can support digestive health, and vitamin B12, which might help with energy levels, are other supplements that might be helpful for ladies over 40. As some supplements may interact with medications or have potential side effects, it is crucial to note that the use of supplements should be addressed with a healthcare professional or a certified dietitian.

Supplements could have a number of advantages, such as:

1. Supporting Overall Health: When a woman's diet has nutrient gaps, supplements can help to fill those gaps, promoting general health and wellbeing. The advantages of supplements can,

however, differ depending on the person and their particular health requirements, it is essential to note.

Furthermore, supplements must be used in conjunction with a healthy diet and way of life; they must not be used in lieu of a diverse and well-balanced diet. Prior to beginning the use of any new supplements, it is always advised to seek the advice of a healthcare professional or a qualified dietitian to make sure they are secure and suitable for the user's requirements.

2.Addressing Specific Nutrients Deficiencies: Specific nutrients that may be missing from a woman's nutrition can be supplied by supplements. For instance, women over 40 may have lower amounts of vitamin B12, which is essential for producing red blood cells and keeping healthy nerve function. This deficit can be treated by taking a vitamin B12 supplement.

Some supplements can help improve the absorption of certain

nutrients. For instance, vitamin D supplements can improve calcium uptake, which is crucial for preserving bone health. Immune function, which is crucial for general health and wellbeing, can be supported by supplements like vitamin C, vitamin D, and zinc. These supplements may be particularly crucial for dieting women over 40 because calorie limitation can impair immune function.

During menopause, older women may experience hormonal changes that raise their risk of developing nutrient deficiencies. These deficiencies can be addressed and overall health supported during this period with the aid of supplements like calcium, vitamin D, and omega-3 fatty acids.

3. Supporting Bone Health: The chance of osteoporosis increases in women over 40, and supplements like calcium, vitamin D, and magnesium can support bone health. These

supplements can be particularly essential for women who are dieting, as weight loss can increase the risk of bone loss. I would advise older women who are dieting to give sufficient dietary intake of calcium, vitamin D, and other bone-supporting nutrients top priority. Supplements can, however, occasionally assist in addressing problems with bone health. For women over 40 dieting to promote bone health, the following supplements may be beneficial:

a. Calcium: To keep healthy bones, women over 40 must consume at least 1,000 milligrams of calcium each day. Supplements can help guarantee appropriate calcium intake if dietary sources are insufficient.

b. Vitamin D: Vitamin D is essential for calcium absorption and bone health. Women over 40 need at least 600-800 IU of vitamin D per day. Vitamin D can be obtained from sunlight, fortified foods, or supplements.

c. Magnesium: Due to its role in the development of bone cells, magnesium is crucial for bone health. Around 320 mg of magnesium are required by women over 40 each day.

d. Vitamin K: Because it aids in the activation of osteocalcin, an enzyme required for bone mineralization, vitamin K is crucial for the health of the bones. About 90 milligrams of vitamin K per day are required for women over 40.

e. Collagen: Protein called collagen makes up a sizable percentage of bone tissue. Collagen supplements could increase bone density and lower injury risk in women over 40.

f. Omega-3 Fatty Acids: With their anti-inflammatory properties, omega-3 fatty acids may help women over 40 lower their chance of bone loss and fractures.

4. Supporting Heart Health: The following particular supplements

may be beneficial for heart health:

a. Omega-3 Fatty Acids: Fatty fish like salmon are a good source of omega-3 fatty acids, which can help to reduce inflammation in the body and possibly reduce the chance of heart disease. If you don't get enough omega-3 fatty acids in your diet, women over 40 may profit from taking a fish oil supplement.

b. Coenzyme Q10 (CoQ10) is an antioxidant that is present in all of the body's cells and is used in the creation of energy. According to some studies, CoQ10 may help lower heart disease risk, particularly in those who take drugs to decrease cholesterol. But this subject requires more study.

c. Vitamin D: Vitamin D is essential for maintaining bone health, but it may also have effects on the heart. Low vitamin D levels have been linked to an increased chance of heart disease, according to some studies. Supplements may be helpful for women over 40 who do not consume enough vitamin D from food and sun exposure.

d.Magnesium is an element that is

essential to the body's many functions, including the maintenance of healthy blood pressure and blood sugar levels. According to some studies, magnesium may help lower the risk of heart disease. A supplement may be helpful for women over 40 who do not consume enough magnesium in their food.

In summary, supplements can be a helpful addition to a healthy diet for women over 40, but they should not be used as a replacement for a balanced and varied diet. Women in this age range may profit from taking supplements that fill in any nutrient gaps in their diet or handle particular health issues. To make sure supplements are secure and suitable for a person's requirements, it's crucial to discuss their use with a medical professional or a registered dietitian.

4.2 Protein Powder

A common dietary supplement that can add another form of protein to your diet is protein powder. For women over 40 who are trying to reduce weight or keep their muscle mass, protein powders can be a beneficial addition to a healthy diet. It becomes more difficult to keep a healthy weight as we age because our bodies naturally lose muscle mass and our metabolic rate slows down. A healthy metabolism and the preservation of muscle mass depend on an adequate protein consumption. Particularly for women who might have difficulty consuming enough protein from whole food sources, protein powders can be a simple and practical method to increase one's protein intake.

When selecting a protein powder, it's crucial to take into account both the protein's quality and any additional components. Whey protein is a well-liked option due to its high quality and quick absorption rate, but people who are lactose sensitive or allergic to dairy products may not be able to use it. For those who prefer a non-dairy source of protein, plant-based protein powders like soy or pea protein are also excellent choices. It's important to consider both the protein's content and any additives when choosing a protein powder. Due to its high quality and speedy absorption, whey protein is a popular choice, but those who are lactose intolerant or averse to dairy products may not be able to use it. Plant-based protein powders like soy or pea protein are also fantastic options for those who prefer a non-dairy form of protein.

The source, grade, and nutritional makeup of the various varieties of protein powder are different. The most popular kinds of protein supplements consist of:

1. Whey Protein: All nine of the necessary amino acids are present in whey protein, which is a milk byproduct and is regarded as a complete

protein. Due to its superior amino acid profile and quick absorption rate, it is a preferred option among athletes and fitness enthusiasts. Protein can aid in reducing hunger and enhancing feelings of fullness because it is more satiating than either fat or carbohydrates. This is particularly crucial for women over 40 who may experience hunger and desires when dieting. Whey protein can help to improve satiety and reduce overeating at meals and snacks.

Protein can be easily and quickly added to meals or treats with whey protein powders without adding a lot of extra calories. In order to increase protein intake without substantially increasing calorie intake, many whey protein powders are low in calories and can be used in recipes like smoothies, protein bars, and protein pancakes.

2.Casein Protein: Casein protein is another type of protein derived from milk. A slow-digesting protein called casein allows for a steady flow of amino acids into the bloodstream. This makes it perfect for use by women over 40 who want to preserve muscle mass and avoid muscle breakdown during prolonged fasting times as a nighttime protein supplement or meal replacement (such as during sleep). Additionally, compared to other proteins like whey protein, casein protein is more satiating. For women over 40 who might have trouble controlling their appetites while dieting, this can help to lessen hunger and desires. Casein protein is a high-quality protein that, like whey protein, includes all of the essential amino acids required for the synthesis of muscle protein. A sufficient protein intake, which includes casein protein, can help improve body composition and keep muscle mass while losing weight.

3.Soy Protein:A complete protein, soy protein is

obtained from soybeans. Because it is a plant-based protein, it is a preferred option for vegetarians and vegans. According to some studies, soy consumption may reduce the chance of developing some cancers, including breast and ovarian cancer. and is complete proteins. It is a popular choice among vegetarians and vegans because it is a plant-based protein source. Soy protein is a high-quality protein that includes all of the necessary amino acids required for the synthesis of muscle protein, just like whey and casein protein. A sufficient protein intake, which includes soy protein, can help improve body composition and keep muscle mass while losing weight.

It has been demonstrated that soy protein has positive impacts on cardiovascular health, such as lowering blood pressure, enhancing lipid profiles, and decreasing inflammation. For women over 40 who have an increased chance of cardiovascular disease, this can be especially crucial. Isoflavones, which are substances found in soy and which have the potential to function as phytoestrogens, can help to regulate hormone levels in women over 40 who may be experiencing menopausal-related hormonal changes. According to some studies, soy consumption may reduce the chance of developing some cancers, including breast and ovarian cancer.

4.Pea Protein: Pea protein, which comes from yellow split peas, is a good source of essential amino acids. It is a good option for people who have food allergies or intolerances because it is hypoallergenic and easily digestible. People who want to increase their protein intake and gain or maintain muscle mass frequently take this supplement. Pea protein can be a particularly useful supplement for dieting older women.

First off, pea protein is a fantastic source of protein for ladies over 40 who might be losing muscle mass as they age. This is due to the fact that pea protein contains a lot of branched-chain amino acids (BCAAs), which are crucial for maintaining and growing muscle. In fact, studies have found that older adults who consume pea protein have thicker, stronger muscles.

Secondly, because pea protein is a complete protein and includes all nine necessary amino acids, it is a good choice for women who follow a plant-based or vegetarian diet. This is crucial because the body cannot produce these amino acids on its own; instead, it must consume them through food.

Thirdly, pea protein is a low-calorie and low-fat supplement that can assist women in obtaining the necessary amounts of protein while avoiding overindulging in calories. Women who are dieting and trying to lose weight or keep their weight within healthy range may find this to be especially helpful.

5. Rice Protein: High in protein: One plant-based protein option with a lot of protein is rice protein. Protein is a vital substance for the body and is crucial for maintaining, repairing, and growing muscles. Rice protein can assist

women over 40 in achieving their objectives of maintaining muscle mass as they age in order to support a healthy metabolism and bone health. Compared to other protein sources like beef and dairy, rice protein is a low-calorie supplement. For women over 40 who are attempting to lose weight or maintain a healthy weight, this makes it a fantastic choice.

Unlike other protein supplements, which can frequently result in bloating and discomfort, rice protein is simple to process. Rice protein is naturally gluten-free, making it a fantastic choice for ladies who have celiac disease or gluten sensitivity.

All of the essential amino acids that the body requires to function correctly are present in rice protein. Because the body cannot produce these amino acids on its own and must acquire them from food sources, this is significant.

6.Hemp Protein: As a complete protein source, hemp protein has all the essential amino acids the body requires to operate properly. Its high protein content makes it a great choice for ladies over 40 who want to support the health and metabolism of their muscles. Fiber-rich hemp protein can make women feel fuller for longer amounts of time and promote healthy digestion. Adequate fiber consumption is crucial for preventing chronic diseases like heart disease and type 2 diabetes, as well as for keeping healthy blood sugar levels.

Given that hemp protein contains few calories, it is a fantastic choice for women over

40 who are trying to slim down or keep a healthy weight. Omega-3 and omega-6 fatty acids, which are important fatty acids, are also abundant in hemp protein. These beneficial fats can promote heart health, lower inflammation, and enhance cognitive function. Hemp protein is a good choice for

women with dietary sensitivities or allergies because it is naturally gluten-free and does not contain common allergens like dairy or soy.

4.2 BCAAs (Branched-Chain Amino Acid)

Leucine, isoleucine, and valine are a trio of essential

amino acids collectively known as BCAAs. The body is unable to produce these amino acids, so they must be consumed through food or supplements. BCAAs could have a number of advantages, such as:

Muscle Mass preservation: Particularly when dieting or losing weight, BCAAs are essential for maintaining and growing muscle. Women over 40 who are dieting to reduce weight or maintain a healthy weight must maintain their muscle mass in order to support a healthy metabolism and keep their physical performance.

1.Reduced Muscle Soreness: Exercise-related muscular soreness and fatigue can be lessened with the aid of BCAAs. Women over 40 who might experience more muscular soreness and fatigue as a result of age-related changes in muscle mass and strength may find this to be helpful.

2. Appetite Control: For ladies over 40 who are attempting to follow a

calorie-restricted diet, BCAAs can help control appetite and lessen cravings.

3. Improved Insulin Sensitivity: With improved insulin sensitivity and muscular glucose uptake, BCAAs can control blood sugar levels and lessen the risk of developing insulin resistance.

4.Energy Production: During times of low energy intake or exercise, BCAAs can be used as a source of energy. This can support healthy metabolism and help women over 40 who are dieting to maintain their current levels of physical exercise.

There are several different BCAA product varieties on the market. BCAAs are most frequently found in free-form amino acids and protein powders. A concentrated form of BCAAs, free-form amino acids are usually taken as supplements. On the other hand, protein powders may contain BCAAs but also other amino acids and minerals. The proportions of the three amino acids should be taken into account when choosing a BCAA supplement. A supplement with a higher ratio of leucine may be more effective for preserving and constructing muscle mass since leucine is usually regarded as the most crucial of the three BCAAs for synthesizing muscle protein.

4.2.1 Free-Form Amino Acid

Free-form amino acids can be a significant addition to a woman's diet, especially when she is on a strict calorie budget or doing a lot of strenuous exercise. Women's muscle mass and strength naturally decrease with age, which can make it more challenging to keep a healthy weight and be active. Additionally, there is a chance of losing muscle mass along with fat during times of dieting, which could be harmful to general health and wellbeing.

During times of calorie restriction or exercise, free-form amino acids can aid in preventing the breakdown of muscle tissue, maintaining muscle mass and strength. This can be crucial for ladies over 40 who might be losing muscle mass as they age. Free-form amino acids can be crucial for other aspects of health in addition to their function in maintaining muscle mass. For instance, some amino acids are necessary for the synthesis of neurotransmitters that have an impact on mood and cognitive ability. A few amino acids also aid in the immune system's operation, wound healing, and other critical bodily procedures.

4.3 Multivitamins

A form of dietary supplement called multivitamins contains a blend of vitamins and minerals. They are made to offer a practical method to guarantee that you are consuming all the vital nutrients your body requires each day. Multivitamins can be a helpful tool for women over 40 who are dieting to help ensure that their nutrient needs are being met, particularly if they are limiting calories or adhering to a specific dietary plan. Women's nutritional requirements can alter as they get older, and they may need more of vitamins and minerals to support their overall health and wellbeing.

Additionally, if you don't eat a range of nutrient-dense foods while dieting, you run the risk of developing nutrient deficiencies. By ensuring that your body receives all the vital vitamins and minerals it needs to function correctly, multivitamins can help to fill in any nutritional gaps. These particular multivitamins become more crucial to women's general health and wellbeing as they get older.

1. Vitamin D: Vitamin D insufficiency is more common in women over 40 and can have negative effects on immune system, bone health, and general

health. Since vitamin D has been associated with lessened fat accumulation, it is also crucial for managing weight.

By improving the body's intake of calcium and phosphorus, vitamin D supports bone health. Women should take extra care to get enough vitamin D to maintain strong bones as they mature because they are more prone to osteoporosis and bone fractures. Maintaining muscular strength is facilitated by vitamin D, which is crucial for women who are losing muscle mass as they age. A sufficient vitamin D intake can enhance general physical function and help avoid falls. Immune system health depends on adequate vitamin D intake. It aids in controlling immune cell production and reaction to infections, which can help fend off chronic illnesses like cancer, autoimmune conditions, and cardiovascular disease.

There is some data that suggests vitamin D may help control mood.

Low vitamin D levels have been linked to an increased chance of anxiety and depression, according to some studies. The control of weight may benefit from vitamin D as well. According to some studies, low levels of vitamin D are linked to higher levels of body fat, while high levels are linked to lower levels of body fat and a reduced risk of obesity. Women's skin becomes less effective at producing vitamin D from sunlight as they mature, making it more challenging to get enough of the vitamin through sun exposure alone.

2. Fatty fish (like salmon and tuna), egg yolks, and fortified foods like

milk and cereal are foods that are excellent sources of vitamin D. However, it can be challenging for some ladies to get enough vitamin D from food alone, so a supplement may be required. For women over 40, 600–800 IU of vitamin D per day is advised, though some specialists advise higher doses for those who are deficient.

3. Vitamin B12: This nutrient is necessary for the synthesis of DNA and the preservation of healthy nerve cells. It's critical to make sure you're getting enough vitamin B12 because as we get older, our bodies become less capable of absorbing it from food.

The generation of red blood cells and the healthy operation of the nervous system both depend on vitamin B12. By aiding in the transformation of food into energy, it also plays a crucial part in the production of energy. Women's systems may become less effective at absorbing and using vitamin B12 as they age, which can result in fatigue and low energy.

Additionally essential for memory and focus, vitamin B12 supports cognitive function. Low vitamin B12 levels have been linked to dementia risk and brain deterioration, according to research. Although the precise mechanism is unclear, some research indicate that vitamin B12 may be important for bone health. Bone fracture and osteoporosis risk are both reportedly raised by low vitamin B12 levels.

There is some data that suggests vitamin B12 may help control mood. Low vitamin B12 levels have been linked to an increased chance of anxiety and depression, according to some studies. Vitamin B12 may also play a role in heart health. Some research has shown that low levels of vitamin B12 are associated with an increased risk of heart disease, although more research is needed to fully understand this relationship.

Foods high in vitamin B12 include dairy, meat,

seafood, poultry, eggs, and other animal products. However, gastrointestinal problems or other factors may make it challenging for some women to absorb vitamin B12 from food. In these circumstances, a supplement might be required to guarantee sufficient consumption. For females over 40, 2.4

micrograms of vitamin B12 daily consumption is advised.

4. Calcium: Calcium is a necessary mineral that is essential for keeping bone health and avoiding osteoporosis, which makes bones brittle and weak. Once a woman turns 40, her body's capacity to absorb calcium declines,

increasing her chance of osteoporosis. Calcium supplementation therefore becomes more crucial for ladies over 40. Since calcium makes up the majority of bones, maintaining healthy bones requires a sufficient calcium intake. The danger of osteoporosis and fractures can be decreased and bone loss can be stopped with calcium supplements.

Muscular cramps and weakness can result from a calcium deficiency because calcium is necessary for healthy muscular function. The danger of muscle-related injuries can be decreased and muscle function can be maintained with the aid of calcium supplements.

Blood pressure is regulated by calcium, and hypertension can be exacerbated by a calcium deficit. Calcium supplements can lower the chance of hypertension and help control blood pressure. A lower chance of cardiovascular disease has been associated with adequate calcium intake. By keeping healthy blood pressure and lowering the risk of heart disease, calcium supplements can support cardiovascular health.

5.Magnesium: Numerous physiological functions, such as muscle and nerve activity, energy metabolism, and bone health, depend on magnesium. Through blood sugar control and inflammation reduction, it may also aid in weight regulation. Magnesium is necessary for healthy bone development and upkeep. Together with calcium and vitamin D, it contributes to maintaining bone health and preventing osteoporosis. By relaxing blood vessels and lowering the chance of hypertension, magnesium helps to regulate blood pressure. Women over 40 who take magnesium supplements can keep healthy blood pressure levels.

Magnesium is crucial for protecting against heart illness and preserving a healthy heart rhythm. Additionally, it aids in enhancing oxygenation and lowering the danger of blood clots. Due to its anti-inflammatory qualities, magnesium can aid in reducing inflammatory processes within the body. For ladies over 40 who may be dealing with joint pain, arthritis, or other inflammatory conditions, this may be helpful. Magnesium helps to control mood and lessen the signs of anxiety and melancholy. Additionally, it supports improved sleep, which is critical for maintaining general physical and mental health.

Magnesium is necessary for healthy muscle activity and can lessen cramping and spasms in the muscles. This is crucial for women over 40 who might be dealing with stiffness and discomfort in their muscles.

6.Omega-3 Fatty Acids: The essential nutrient omega-3 fatty acids is crucial for keeping good health and preventing chronic diseases. By bringing down blood pressure, reducing inflammation, and lowering triglycerides, omega-3 fatty acids can help lower the chance of heart disease. Omega-3 fatty acids are a crucial component of a woman's diet because women over 40 have an increased chance of developing heart disease.

Omega-3 fatty acids are essential for preserving cognitive

ability and brain wellness. According to studies, omega-3 fatty acids can assist older adults with their memory and lower their risk of cognitive decline. Omega-3 fatty acids have anti-inflammatory properties that can help women over 40 who may be having age-related joint issues lessen joint pain and stiffness. The risk of age-related macular degeneration, the primary cause of blindness in older adults, may be decreased by omega-3 fatty acids, which are crucial for maintaining eye health. The risk of age-related macular degeneration, the primary cause of blindness in older adults, may be decreased by omega-3 fatty acids, which are crucial for maintaining eye health.

In women over 40, omega-3 fatty acids may lessen the intensity of menopause symptoms like hot flashes and night sweats.

4.4 Choosing Supplements Wisely

Making the best decisions when it comes to supplements can be difficult, particularly for dieting ladies over 40. You can follow these actions to make wise decisions:

1. Prior to selecting supplements, it's essential to ascertain your nutritional

requirements. Take into account your age, gender, nutrition, lifestyle, and any medical conditions or prescription drugs you might be taking. Your nutrient requirements can be ascertained with the assistance of a certified dietitian or a physician.

2. After identifying your nutritional requirements, choose supplements that specifically target those requirements. In order to support bone health, for instance, you may profit from taking a calcium and vitamin D supplement if you do not consume enough of these nutrients through your diet.

3. Look for quality brands: Pick an organization with a solid reputation for creating vitamins of the highest caliber. Select goods that have undergone testing from third parties like the US Pharmacopeia (USP), ConsumerLab, or NSF International.

4. Observe labels closely: Make sure to

thoroughly study the labels and select supplements that offer the adequate intake (AI) or recommended daily allowance (RDA) for the particular nutrient. Supplements with high concentrations of any one nutrient should be avoided as they may be detrimental.

5. A healthcare expert should be consulted if you are taking any medications to make sure there are no potential interactions between the supplements you are taking and the medications you are taking.

6. Supplements that guarantee quick or miraculous results

should be avoided because the claims made for them are frequently too good to be true. Stick to dietary supplements that have been proven successful in clinical trials and supported by science.

Chapter Five

5.0 Staying On Track And Adapting To Changes

It is very important to know that every person's body is different, it's essential to keep in mind that you should always speak with a healthcare provider before making any major dietary or exercise changes.

Women's bodies alter as they get older, which can

make it harder to keep up a healthy weight. A slower metabolism, a loss of muscle mass, and hormonal adjustments that may lead to weight increase are some of these changes. Women over a certain age may also be taking medications or coping with other health problems that could affect their weight. In order to maintain their general health and wellbeing, it is crucial for women over a certain age to remain on track with their dieting goals. A nutritious diet can aid in the management or prevention of persistent illnesses like diabetes, heart disease, and some types of cancer.

Here are some pointers to help ladies over a certain age adjust to changes and maintain their dieting objectives:

1. Focus on nutrient-dense foods: As we age, our bodies require more nutrients to remain healthy. Eat a range of fruits, vegetables, whole grains, lean proteins, and healthy fats as your main focus.

2. Watch your serving sizes because as we age, our metabolism may not burn as many calories as

it once did. Pay attention to portion sizes and try to consume just enough to feel satisfied rather than stuffing yourself.

3. Exercise frequently to keep muscle mass and speed up your metabolism. Try to exercise for at least 30 minutes, most days of the week, at a moderate effort.

4. Keep yourself hydrated because thirst and confusion from dehydration can affect your appetite and dietary preferences. If you are active or live in a hot environment, consume more water than the recommended minimum of 8 cups per day.

5. Get enough rest because insufficient slumber can interfere with the hormones that control appetite and metabolism. Sleep for 7-8 hours every night.

6. Seek assistance: Changing your nutrition can be difficult, particularly if you have other health problems. To assist you in staying

on track, ask your friends, family, or a healthcare provider for assistance.

In conclusion, women over a certain age should keep a healthy diet to manage or prevent chronic conditions and to maintain overall health and well-being. Although adjusting to changes in metabolism and hormones can be difficult, maintaining your weight loss objectives is possible with a focus on nutrient-dense foods, portion control, regular exercise, hydration, enough sleep, and support.

5.1 Staying Motivated

Everybody needs to stay motivated to keep up a healthy diet, but ladies over 40 may find it especially difficult to do so due to the following reasons:

1. Hormonal changes: Hormonal changes in women over 40, such as menopause, can have an

impact on their temperament, energy level, and metabolism. Maintaining an active lifestyle and a healthy diet may become more challenging as a result of these shifts.

2.Numerous women over 40 may lead busy lives that involve balancing job, family, and other responsibilities. It can be difficult to find the time to make wholesome meals and exercise.

3.Metabolic rate: Women's metabolic rates tend to slow down as they get older, making it easier to acquire weight and harder to lose it. This can make maintaining a healthy diet and exercise regimen discouraging.

4. Social pressure: Women over 40 may also experience social pressure to look a certain way, which can be demotivating. They might experience pressure to keep looking young, which is challenging to do with just diet and exercise.

5. Health problems: As women get older, they may also experience health problems that make it harder to follow a healthy diet and exercise regimen. For instance, it might be challenging to exercise if you have arthritis or joint discomfort.

Women over 40 can overcome these difficulties and accomplish their health goals by being aware of these issues and putting strategies like realistic goal-setting, finding a support system, and being consistent into practice and the result that follows would be mind blowing. A comprehensive explanation of the strategies to employ to achieve desirable results:

1.Recognize the rationale behind the plan. It's crucial to know your motivations before starting any diet or exercise regimen. Maintaining a healthy weight, preventing chronic illnesses, or improving general health and wellbeing may be the driving forces behind women over 40. Understanding the motivation's underlying causes can help you maintain your commitment to your objectives and keep your concentration.

2. Goal setting: Setting attainable and practical objectives is essential for maintaining motivation. Goals for women over 40 should

take into account their current physical condition and way of living. It's essential to keep in mind that development might be gradual and that obstacles might appear. However, women over 40 can maintain motivation and recognize small accomplishments along the way by establishing realistic goals.

3. Find a system of assistance: The key to maintaining motivation is having a support system. Support for women over 40 can be obtained from family, friends, or online communities. In trying times, a support network

can offer inspiration, responsibility, and drive.

4. Be Consistent: Success in keeping a healthy diet depends on consistency. Women who are over 40 should make it a habit to consume well and exercise. This entails figuring out how to work healthy eating and exercise into everyday schedules. These

routines will eventually become second nature, making it simpler to remain on course.

5.1.1 Accountable

In order to keep a healthy diet and reach their weight loss goals, accountability is a crucial component. Accountability means accepting responsibility for one's actions and holding oneself and others responsible for achieving particular objectives. In the setting of dieting for women over 40, accountability can be useful in the following ways:

1. Accountability to oneself: Women over 40 who want to drop a few pounds or keep up a healthy diet should start by establishing concrete

objectives and monitoring their development. This can be done by maintaining a food diary, using a weight loss app, or simply writing down objectives and progress in a journal. Women over 40 can hold themselves accountable and alter their diet as necessary by monitoring their food and weight.

2.Accountability to a partner or friend: Having a partner or friend who can hold you responsible for your eating and exercise habits can be beneficial for women over 40. By keeping track of their progress and assisting them in setting sensible goals, this person can offer them encouragement, support, and help them stay on course.

3. Accountability to a nutritionist or coach: Women over 40 who work with one have access to a professional who can assist them in developing a personalized diet plan, setting objectives, and offering support and

accountability. A nutritionist or coach can also educate women over 40 about healthy eating practices and assist them in making long-lasting lifestyle adjustments.

4. Group accountability: Women over 40 who take part in a support group or weight reduction program can

gain from meeting people who share their goals. This group can give support and motivation as well as a feeling of community and accountability.

Overall, accountability is an essential element of dieting for women over 40. Women over 40 can stay on track with their diet and reach their weight reduction objectives by taking responsibility for their actions and asking for assistance. Accountability can help women over 40 develop healthy habits that can last a lifetime, whether it's through self-monitoring, support from a partner or friend, working with a nutritionist or coach, or engaging in a group.

5.2 Tracking Progress

Any objective, such as losing weight or keeping up a healthy diet, can be accomplished with tracking progress. Here are a few strategies for monitoring your weight-loss progress:

- Keeping a food diary: A popular and useful method for monitoring weight loss success when dieting is keeping a food diary. Simply put, a food journal is a list of all the food and beverages you consume each day. This is how it goes:

a. Start by selecting a strategy: To keep track of your meals and beverages, you can use a journal, a smartphone tool, or a website. Pick a technique that is simple and handy for you to use on a regular basis.

b.Keep track of everything you consume: Note everything you consume, including the quantity and time of day, in a written journal. Include as much information as you can, such as the food's variety and brand, the quantity eaten, and any toppings or condiments you used.

c. Be truthful: It's critical to be truthful when logging your meals and beverages. Write it down even if you consume an unhealthy snack or consume too much food at a dinner. You can then spot trends in your eating behavior and pinpoint areas that need development.

d. Regularly review your food diary and ruminate on what you ate and how you felt. Make time each day to do this. In order to better, look for trends or triggers that contributed to your unhealthy eating patterns.

e. Make adjustments: Adjust your diet as necessary in light of your evaluation. This could entail limiting certain food categories, selecting healthier snacks, or reducing portion sizes.

You can better understand your eating patterns and improve your diet by maintaining a food diary. According to research, keeping a food diary can increase your awareness of unhealthy eating patterns, aid in weight loss, and give you a feeling of accountability. It can also assist you in identifying patterns in your eating behavior that may be causing weight increase or other health issues, such as consuming an excessive amount of sugar or high-calorie foods. In conclusion, keeping a food journal is a useful way to monitor your progress while dieting and can encourage you to choose healthier options in order to reach your weight loss objectives.

2. Use a scale: When attempting to improve your health and fitness, taking measurements is an essential way to monitor your progress. More information on taking and tracking data can be found here:

Waist Circumference: Your waist circumference can serve as a gauge for your level of abdominal fat, which has been linked to a higher chance of conditions like heart disease, diabetes, and some types of cancer. Wrap a tape measure snugly (but not too tightly) around your waist at your abdominal button to get your waist measurement. Keep note of the measurement over time to determine whether it is decreasing by writing it down in inches or centimeters.

- Body weight: This quantity may serve as a sign of broader alterations in body composition. While it's important to keep in mind that changes in body weight can occur due to things like water retention and muscle growth, monitoring it over time can still reveal progress. Use a scale to weigh yourself at the same time every day, ideally in the morning and without any clothing on, to determine your body weight. Keep note of the measurement over time by recording it.

- Body fat percentage: When compared to body weight alone, this measurement can provide a more accurate image of your body composition. Body fat proportion can be determined using a variety of techniques, such as bioelectrical impedance analysis or skinfold calipers. Even if your body weight remains constant over time, tracking your body fat percentage can help you see changes in your body composition.

It's crucial to be consistent with how and when you collect your measurements when keeping track of them. Measurements should be taken on a frequent basis, such as weekly or monthly, and should be recorded in a journal or a mobile app. You can use this to track patterns and improvements over time. Keep in mind that progress is not always straightforward and that there may be ups and downs along the road. Tracking your metrics, however, can support your motivation and goal-focused behavior.

3. Taking progress photos: Taking progress pictures as you go along with your diet is a great method to monitor your physical changes. You may not immediately observe changes in your body's composition and shape when you look in the mirror, but these photos can help you do that. Wear form-fitting clothing that makes it

possible to see your body shape plainly when taking progress photos. Take three pictures: one frontal, one sidelong, and one backward. These pictures can be taken by yourself in a full-length mirror or by a third party.

To track changes over time, it's critical to take progress pictures frequently, ideally every two to four weeks. You'll be able to see how your body has changed when you compare your pictures side by side, and this can be a strong motivator to continue.

You can use a measuring tape to take measurements of your physique in addition to taking pictures. You can use this to keep tabs on changes to your waistline and hips, for example. Keep in mind that losing weight and changing your body take time, so be patient and persistent in your efforts.

4. Take body measurements: As a woman over 40 on a diet, taking body measurements is

another method to monitor your progress. Body measurements can give you a more accurate image of how your body is changing than the scale, which is still a useful tool. Here are some pointers for measuring your body:

Use a measuring tape: To record your measurements, use a soft, flexible measuring tape. These are available online or at the majority of craft shops.

- Measurements should be taken at the same time every week; ideally, this should be in the morning before ingesting or drinking anything.

- Take measurements of particular body parts, including your waist, hips, thighs, arms, and torso. Keep a record of these numbers over time by writing them down.

- When taking measurements, make sure the measuring tape is level and snug but not too rigid. Measure in the same location each time.

- Don't give up: Keep in mind that it's acceptable

if your body measurements don't change every week. The results will arrive if you are persistent and patient with your diet and exercise program.

Regular body measurements allow you to monitor changes in particular body parts and identify success that may not be visible on the scale. This may be a great method to maintain your motivation and progress toward your weight loss objectives.

5. Track your energy levels and moods: An often-overlooked aspect of monitoring diet progress is keeping note of your energy and mood. However, doing so can help you understand how your diet is affecting your general well-being. Following are some pointers

for monitoring your vitality and mood:

Keep a diary: Write down your daily feelings, including how you're feeling emotionally and physiologically. Take note of your mood, your level of vitality, and any cravings you may be having.

6. Be mindful of your body: Pay focus to your feelings throughout the day by

tuning into your body. Do certain meals make you feel lethargic afterwards? Do you feel more energized following a certain dinner or snack? Utilize this knowledge to modify your diet and workout regimen.

7. Analyze patterns: Look for patterns in your diary as you read it frequently. Are there particular days or times of the week when you

regularly lack energy? Do some meals give you more energy or make you feel less full?

8. Celebrate minor victories: If you notice an improvement in your mood or energy level, do so. They may serve as a strong source of motivation.

You can better grasp how your diet is affecting your

general well-being by keeping track of your energy levels and mood. This knowledge can assist you in making changes to your diet and exercise program and can serve as a strong source of inspiration as you strive to reach your weight reduction objectives.

5.4 Adjusting Diet And Exercise Routine

Women's bodies alter as they age, which may have an impact on their nutritional requirements. For women over 40, dieting can be a healthy way to manage their weight and keep good health, but it's crucial to adopt a sustainable and balanced approach to dieting. Women over 40 who want to lose weight should take the following important aspects into account when changing their diets:

1. Choose foods that are rich in nutrients because women over 40 need more nutrients to support their aging bodies. Their diet should be built around nutrient-dense foods like fruits, veggies, whole grains, lean proteins, and healthy fats. These

foods offer vital vitamins, minerals, fiber, and antioxidants that can lower the chance of developing chronic illnesses like cancer, diabetes, and heart disease.

2.Boost your protein intake: Women's bodies naturally lose muscle mass as they mature, which can slow metabolism and increase the risk of weight gain. Women over 40 should strive to eat more high-quality protein sources, such as seafood, poultry, eggs, beans, and nuts, in order to help combat this. Additionally, it can help them feel satiated and full all day long.

3. Reduce your intake of processed foods and added sugars because they can cause inflammation, weight increase, and other health issues. Women over 40 should make an effort to reduce their consumption of these foods and instead concentrate on whole, unadulterated foods.

4.Keep hydrated: Dehydration is a frequent issue as we age because our bodies may become less adept at maintaining fluid balance. Women over 40 should try to consume at least 8 to 10 glasses of water daily and stay away from alcohol and sweetened beverages.

5. Think about supplements: Although whole foods are always the best source of nutrients, women over 40 may profit from taking specific supplements to support their general health. Omega-3 fatty acids, vitamin D, and calcium supplements may be especially crucial for cardiac and bone health.

6. Consult a registered dietitian: A registered dietitian can assist women over the age of 40 in developing a customized nutrition plan that takes into consideration their unique requirements, preferences, and health objectives. They can aid in tracking success and offer advice on

developing healthy eating habits.

5.4.1 Exercise Routine

Exercise is crucial for keeping good health, particularly as we get older. Regular exercise can increase cardiovascular health, lower the chance of chronic diseases, increase bone density, and improve overall quality of life.

Regular physical activity contributes to general health and wellbeing. Exercise can enhance mental health, lower the chance of chronic diseases, improve cardiovascular health, and manage weight. Here is a thorough description of a workout regimen along with some suggestions for various exercises:

1.Cardiovascular exercise: Any action that speeds up your heart rate and breathing rate is considered cardiovascular exercise, also referred to as cardio or aerobic exercise. Exercise of this kind is crucial for preserving cardiovascular health, enhancing stamina, and burning calories. Cardiovascular activities come in a wide variety of forms, such as walking, jogging, cycling, swimming, dancing, and more. Adults should perform at least 150 minutes of moderate-intensity or 75 minutes of vigorous-intensity cardiovascular activity each week, according to the American Heart Association. Exercise of a moderate level causes you to breathe more heavily than usual, but you are still able to speak normally. Exercises that fall under the category of moderate intensity include brisk strolling, level-surface cycling, and water aerobics. A discussion is challenging while engaging in vigorous exercise because your breathing is moving quickly.

Exercises that require a high level of intensity include sprinting, intense cycling, and jumping rope. It's essential to remember that everyone's level of fitness is unique, so your age, fitness level, and health status may all affect how much cardiovascular exercise is right for you. If you've never worked out before, it's a good idea to start out gently and build up the length and intensity of your workouts over time. If it's more convenient for you, you can also spread out your exercise into smaller sessions throughout the day.

Cardiovascular exercise has advantages for mental health as well as bodily health. Cardiovascular exercise can enhance mood, increase energy levels, and aid with stress and anxiety reduction. Overall, a healthy living includes cardiovascular exercise in your regimen. To create a sustainable habit, it is advised to choose activities you will appreciate and be able to maintain over time.

Recommended cardiovascular exercises:

- Brisk walking: A low-impact

cardiovascular exercise that is simple to include in a daily practice is brisk walking. Additionally, it is fantastic for boosting bone density and lowering the chance of chronic illnesses.

- Swimming: Swimming is a low-impact cardiovascular activity that can help increase strength, flexibility, and endurance. As the buoyancy of the water lessens stress on the joints, it's also a fantastic choice for women who have joint pain or other injuries.

- Running and jogging: Running and jogging are high-impact exercises that can increase cardiovascular stamina and help you lose weight. Women with joint issues, however, might find it inappropriate.

- Cycling: Cycling is a low-impact activity that can strengthen your legs and cardiovascular system. On a stationary cycle, you can do it both inside and outside.

- Dancing: Dancing is an enjoyable activity that can help you lose weight and improve your cardiovascular health. It can be carried out at home or in a group situation.

- Strength training: Utilizing weights, resistance bands, or bodyweight exercises to increase strength and muscular mass is known as strength training, also referred to as resistance training or weight training. Strength training helps to improve bone density, which lowers the chance of osteoporosis, and maintain or increase muscle mass, which naturally declines with aging in women over 40. At least two sessions of strength exercise per week are advised for women over 40. It's crucial to start with lighter weights when starting a strength training program and to concentrate on correct form and technique. As you get stronger, gradually raise the weight or resistance. Exercises for strength training can target particular muscle areas, like squats, lunges, push-ups, and shoulder presses. All of the main muscle groups, including the legs, back, chest, shoulders, arms, and core, should be worked.

2. Strength training has many physical advantages, but it can also help with

weight loss and general health by enhancing body composition and metabolism. It's crucial to remember that for best outcomes, strength training should be combined with aerobic exercise and a balanced diet.

Recommend Strength Training Exercise

- Squats - Squats are a compound exercise that work the glutes, quads, and hamstrings as well as other muscles in the lower body.
- Lunges - Lunges help increase balance and stability while targeting the same muscle areas as squats.

- Deadlifts: Deadlifts are a great workout for strengthening the entire body, especially the lower back and hamstrings.

- Push-ups - Push-ups are a simple exercise that can be modified to suit a variety of fitness levels and target the chest, arms, and shoulders.

- Aided pull-ups or pull-ups: Pull-ups are a difficult workout that strengthens the shoulders, biceps, and back. Resistance bands or an assisted pull-up equipment can be used by women who aren't yet able to perform pull-ups on their own.
- Planks: Planks enhance stability and balance

while helping to develop core strength.

3.Flexibility and balance exercises: Our muscles, tendons, and ligaments typically lose some of their elasticity as we age, rendering them less flexible. The joints may become rigid and have less range of motion as a result, making daily tasks more difficult. Additionally, as we age, our balance may also deteriorate, raising the risk of injuries and crashes. Exercises for flexibility and balance can help to increase flexibility, decrease stiffness, and improve general physical performance. The following are some activities that may be helpful:

• Yoga: Yoga incorporates physical postures, breathing techniques, and meditation in its mind-body discipline. As well as lowering tension and anxiety, it can aid in strengthening, flexibility, and balance.

- Pilates: Pilates is a low-impact exercise method that emphasizes balance, flexibility, and core muscle. It is a fantastic choice for enhancing posture and easing back discomfort because it calls for precise movements and controlled breathing.

- Tai Chi: Tai Chi is a traditional Chinese exercise that entails deep breathing and slow, flowing motions. It can help with stress relief and cerebral clarity, as well as with balance, flexibility, and coordination.

- Stretching: Stretching can help increase joint suppleness and range of motion, making it simpler to carry out daily tasks. All main muscular groups, including the hamstrings, calves, chest, shoulders, and back, should be stretched.

5.4 Adapting to Changes and Setbacks

Every health path requires adjustment to obstacles and changes, even for women over 40 who are on a diet and taking supplements. Here are some pointers on how to modify your diet and supplement regimen in the event of changes or setbacks:

1.Set achievable and practical goals: When establishing objectives for your diet and supplement regimen, make sure they are both. Setting unattainable goals can cause frustration and a feeling of failure, which makes it harder to bounce back from setbacks.

2.Follow your development: Keep a record of your accomplishments to spur on your motivation and spot potential areas for improvement. In a journal or with a mobile tool, you can keep account of your dietary intake, physical activity, and supplement usage.

3.Be adaptable: As your body and habits change, you may need to occasionally modify your diet and supplement regimen. Be flexible when it comes to altering your supplement regimen, whether that means upping or lowering your dosage or switching to a different kind.

4. If you experience a setback or lapse in your supplement or nutrition regimen, don't give up. Instead, see it as a chance to improve by learning from it.

5. Don't be afraid to ask friends, family, or a medical professional for assistance. Having a support structure can

assist you in remaining driven and responsible.

6. Finally, maintain your positive attitude and concentrate on your accomplishments and development rather than any setbacks. Celebrate your accomplishments and use them as inspiration to keep pursuing your health objectives.

Be patient and kind to yourself along the way, and keep in mind that adjusting to changes and setbacks is a normal part of any path toward better health. You can maintain a healthy diet and supplement regimen and reach your health goals with patience and persistence.